HOW TO GET RID OF ACNE

THE ESSENTIAL GUIDE TO GETTING RID OF ACNE

Table of Contents

INTRODUCTION

Are you battling acne? Then put your trust in these 5 best home remedies for pimples.

If you have acne, stop wasting money on expensive creams and gels. Instead, try these pimple home remedies.

Isn't a pimple unquestionably the most dreadful blemish on the face? We all want flawless skin that is free of acne, dark circles, and other unsightly flaws.

But the worst part about acne is that when one zit disappears, it is quickly replaced by another, leaving behind unwanted redness and acne scars.

Of course, there are numerous products on the market that claim to provide the best acne treatment—but in most cases, these are just claims. And don't even get me started on the side effects.

As a result, we offer the ideal solution to your acne problem: home remedies for pimples.

Did you know that the best treatment for pimples on your face can be found right in your own home? Still not convinced? Then take a look at these effective home remedies for pimples:

➢ CHAPTER 1

Lemon Juice and Aloe Vera

Acne draws your attention when you look in the mirror, and it is annoying. According to a 2014 study published in the Journal of Dermatological Treatment, the antibacterial properties of aloe-Vera can help to reduce bacteria. Not to mention that aloe Vera is soothing and cooling when applied to the skin, which can help to reduce the redness and inflammation caused by

pimples.

To use, combine a tablespoon of freshly

scooped aloe Vera gel with a teaspoon

of lemon juice. Apply the mixture to

your face and rinse after 15 minutes.

➢CHAPTER 2

Yogurt and yeast

If you have oily skin and are prone to acne, a yeast-yogurt mask can help. It's the ideal treatment for clear, glowing skin. Yeast is naturally purifying, and when combined with the antibacterial and antifungal properties of yogurt, it can help to reduce pimples.

Here's how to use it: Combine half a tbsp yogurt and half a tablespoon of instant yeast. Allow this to sit on your face and neck for 20 minutes. Use warm water to wash your face and moisturize as usual.

➢CHAPTER 3

Baking soda and apple cider vinegar

Consider apple cider vinegar to be the "Shakalaka-Boom-Boom" magic pencil that only works to kill pimples! According to a study published in the International Journal of Cosmetic Science, acetic acid

The bacteria that causes acne, is killed by oily, lactic, and citric acid. The good news is that apple cider vinegar contains all of these nutrients.

Here's how to make it: Combine 1 tsp organic apple cider vinegar, 2 tsp water, and 3 tsp baking soda. Apply the solution to your zits. After 20 minutes, wash it off.

Apple cider vinegar is beneficial to the skin.

➢CHAPTER 4

Honey and turmeric

We are all aware that turmeric or haldi can provide us with glowing skin. But did you know that turmeric can also be used to treat acne? Turmeric's polyphenols and cur cumin are excellent for treating inflammatory conditions such as acne.

➢**CHAPTER 5**

Whites of eggs

If you believe that eggs can only be used to bake cakes, you are mistaken. There are numerous advantages to using egg white face masks. They are high in vitamins and proteins and help to regulate sebum production, making your skin less oily. Less oil means less acne.

Here's how to use it: whisk together 1

egg white and 1/2 teaspoon garlic paste.

Apply the mixture to your face for 15

minutes and then wash it off.

➢CHAPTER 6

HOW TO GET RID OF BLACK HEADS

Blackheads are small bumps that appear on your skin due to clogged hair follicles. These bumps are called blackheads because the surface looks dark or black. They appear on other body parts too; the chest, back, neck, arms and shoulders.

Some factors can increase your chances

of developing blackheads and acne,

including:

> Irritation of the hair follicles when

dead skin cells don't shed on a

regular basis.

> Undergoing hormonal changes that

cause an increase in oil production

during the teen years, during

menstruation, or while taking birth

control pills.

➤ Producing too much body oil

➤ Taking certain drugs, such as
corticosteroids, lithium, or
androgens

Most people believe that what you eat
or drink can affect acne. Dairy products
and foods that increase blood sugar
levels, such as carbohydrates, may play
a part in triggering acne, but researchers

aren't convinced that there's a strong connection.

TREATMENTS

➢PRESCRIPTION MEDICATIONS

If over the counter treatment doesn't improve your acne, your doctor may suggest that you use stronger prescription medications.

Medications that contain vitamin A keeps plug from forming in the hair follicles and promote more rapid turnover of skin cells.

➢ OVER-THE-COUNTER [OTC] TREATMENTS

Many acne medications are available at drug and grocery stores and online without prescription. These medications are available in cream, gel and pad form and are put directly on your skin. The drugs contain benzoyl peroxide, resorcinol and salicylic acid. They work by killing bacteria, drying, excess oil

and forcing skin to shed dead skin cells.

➤**MANUAL REMOVAL**

Dermatologists or specially trained skin

care professionals use a special

instrument called a round loop extractor

to remove the plug causing the

blackhead.

➤

➢LASER AND LIGHT THERAPY

Laser and light therapies use tiny beams of intense light to decrease oil production or kill bacteria. Both lasers and light beams reach below the surface of the skin to treat blackheads and acne without damaging the top layers of the skin.

HOME REMEDIES

➢ USE OF BAKING SODA AND WATER

You can get rid of the tricky, firm blackheads using this home remedy.

Oatmeal scrub: make a scrub with plain yoghurt, half lemon juice, I tablespoon oatmeal. Leave the scrub for 15 minutes on your face and rinse it off with lukewarm water.

➢CLAY

Masks made from fuller's earth and kaolin clay, when used regularly on the face can help clear out the pores. This will eventually get rid of blackheads and make the skin smooth.

➤STEAMING

Steaming the face makes the skin sweat, which in turn helps to clear out toxins from within. It also softens the pores, making the stubborn blackheads easier to work upon and remove.

If you read this book to the end, I'm sure you now know how to get rid of acne, blackheads and pimples at home

with less cost and stress.